T0132095

The Everyday Bodysmith LLC

A Practical and Progressive Guide to the Bodysmithing Philosophy

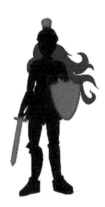

HEATHER ANN NOONAN LMP

Senior Editor Laurie Whittington

AuthorHouse™
1663 Liberty Drive
Bloomington, IN 47403
www.authorhouse.com
Phone: 833-262-8899

Because of the dynamic nature of the Internet, any web addresses or links contained in this book may have changed
since publication and may no longer be valid. The views expressed in this work are solely those of the author and do not
necessarily reflect the views of the publisher, and the publisher hereby disclaims any responsibility for them.

Any people depicted in stock imagery provided by Getty Images are models,
and such images are being used for illustrative purposes only.
Certain stock imagery © Getty Images.

Scripture taken from the Holy Bible, New International Version®. Copyright © 1973, 1978,
1984 Biblica. Used by permission of Zondervan. All rights reserved.

This book is printed on acid-free paper.

ISBN: 978-1-6655-5609-5 (sc)
ISBN: 978-1-6655-5610-1 (e)

Library of Congress Control Number: 2022906059

Print information available on the last page.

Published by AuthorHouse 04/07/2022

authorHOUSE®

Contents

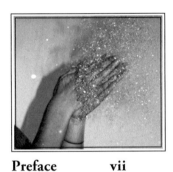

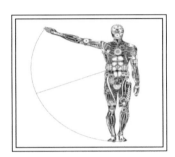

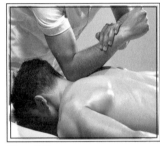

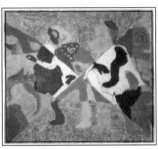

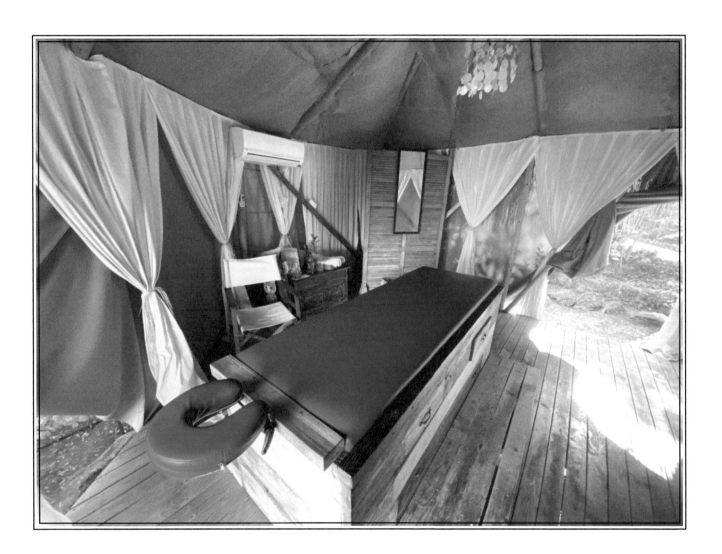

Preface

This guide is divided into three parts; Prep Work, Massages and Treatments, and Core Insights concerning the BodySmith Philosophy.

Part I dives into Body Mechanics, wearing a Mask, and the BodySmith Pressure Scale, where the work starts.

The services, Part II, are quite progressive. Entailed are the names of massages and their designated techniques and purposes. These treasured skills should not be used out of context. The collection will become easily discernible for anyone who follows the guidelines and philosophy.

With careful consideration, a BodySmith will assess, evaluate, and discuss which massage would be most effective with the client and provide the freedom to ask questions. These interactions will pleasantly surprise the inductive reasoning skills, improving confidence to represent bodysmithing.

The third part of this guide provides Core Insight with Body Armor, the origination of our divine calling as BodySmiths, and The Temple needing help with its Armor. In order to have compassion and kindness in a practice, it's imperative to see every person as having invisible Armor. A BodySmith discerns more than what meets the eyes. Observational perception combined with spiritual discernment is a key piece to working with the human body.

Enjoy this compilation of wisdom for the love of bodysmithing!

Cheers and God Bless, to wellness recovery and peace of mind.

Heather Noonan, President of The BodySmith

Introduction

Bodysmithing Today and Philosophy

Message Therapy: a necessity for some, a treat for others. Cultivating itself among America within the past 20 years, massage has blossomed from a luxury to a weekly need.

Massage therapy can be divided into many categories: Tai, Sports, Pediatric, Hot/Cold stone, Deep Tissue, Lomi Lomi, Swedish, and Medical. Often therapists find a niche and stick with it. They own a specialty and work on creating a 'Need' for their service. Or, they work for someone else who created that 'Need' and is hopefully enjoying being an employee.

Hospitals, Chiropractic and Physical Therapist offices, Day Spas, Retreat Centers, Massage Chains, they all employ massage with a preconceived notion of what massage should be, pertaining to their company's service. Having practiced the art of massage in all of the above, it's been valuable to learn skills catering to specific specialties and persons.

Bodysmithing is a developing concept on the tails of blacksmithing or gunsmithing. The title or business name of the BodySmith is not new. This guide however, is a new practical and progressive approach to bodysmithing, detailing carefully determined methods and intentions derived from my many experiences.

The philosophy behind bodysmithing entails the what, how and why? The 'How and Why' is addressed in Part III: Core Insights, The Armor and Temple chapters. You can skip there now if you are so intrigued!

Why am I using my over 16 years of acquired and refined massage skills to help people? In short, human bodies don't work the way they should and I want to help improve their quality of life through bodysmithing. My specialties are a stepping stone to wellness, recovery and peace of mind. I love encouraging people to take their overall health into their own hands and live their best life possible.

Bodysmithing takes a body that doesn't quite work the way it should, be it from injury, stress, work, sports, pregnancy, accidents, etc., and helps the person repair it. By analyzing body/muscle disorders, I use my extensive experience of working alongside Chiropractors, PT's, day spas, teaching and learning under a Russian

Medical Doctor, and a Pediatric healer, Rolfer, to help the client help themselves.

Bodysmithing is like blacksmithing. Dennis Davidson, a forger in the gorge, quotes below what blacksmithing is.

Just as "a blacksmith takes metal to restore or create something new", a BodySmith takes what they are given from a person and uses this practical and progressive guide to be a part of restoring and improving a person's quality of life.

On a very important side note, I am also sharing my wisdom because as a BodySmith, I am very concerned about the abuse heaped on many great massage therapists. Many work 8 hours a day, 5 days a week using skills far above their pay.

There should be a standard of what massage is in its proper context, with its proper wage. With my philosophy, I believe that the ***massage therapy standard will be set,*** esteemed to its highest, eventually, hiring those that value the art of true, unblemished, wise and qualitative massage.

I pray that I can see a new generation practicing massage therapists become BodySmiths. Massage in this practical and progressive program is not based on intuition. Nor is based on fluff and buff. While there is credibility in being able to sense what's causing the discomfort in a muscle or just giving a massage well, there is an elevated respect among physicians, insurance companies, and clients when they know, that

you know, why you are doing every single technique on a body during a session. (A good gardener doesn't just love the garden. They also have to hate the weeds).

Thank you for allowing me to teach you, opening your mind and senses to the new world of bodysmithing! May your practice abound with good testimonies that encourage those who are looking for a lighthouse in these dark times. And, for those who are on the receiving end, remember that the real journey to healing is in your dedication and personal intention all day, every day, to getting better and feeling your best!

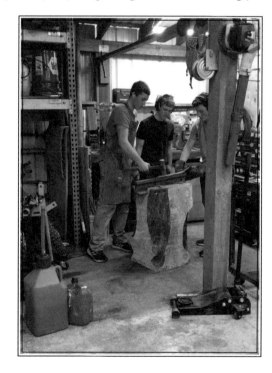

PART I:

PREPWORK

The BodySmith Endurance, Stamina, and Perseverance

BodyMechanics

'Exercise is a celebration of what your body can do, not a punishment for what you ate.' Your finished work is as good as your tools; ask any mechanic. A BodySmith is represented in how they take care of themselves. From the first impression whether you are healthy or not, to the tiny details of having your toenails trimmed and cleaned, showing without words that we care about our own health and peace of mind causes people to believe and trust that you will take care of them.

A daily intention to strengthen your muscles or relax them if you work all day is a necessity. It is vital to wake up at 6am, jog a mile or two, stretch, shower and arrive at the studio 15 min. before a morning appointment. This awakening of your body, enables you to create an atmosphere of growth during the session. If you have warmed up your mind and body, you are ahead of the game.

A good day begins the night before. If you go to bed at 3am, don't brag about it during a session. The client doesn't want to pay for you to play and hobble into work tired and hung over. This routine is Unacceptable. A BodySmith never treats their body this way and should promote their temple (body) with its endurance, stamina and perseverance. Furthermore, Self Control is an attractive attribute easily seen and highly sought after.

Bodysmiths show they care about themselves in such a way without words, that it invites and intrigues a person to ask what they do need to investigate on their own health journey.

Something little and silly but I like to have my toenails painted because people are staring at them for 30-40 min during a massage.

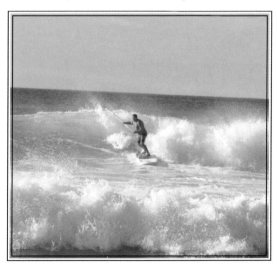

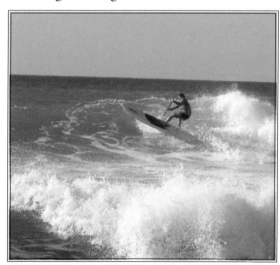

Taking care of just a little detail, such as keeping clean toenails, subconsciously relays to the client that I take care of the little details, so I must pay attention to the big details they are telling me about before a session.

After 16 years of practice, and having incredible teachers and fellow bodyworkers who would correct, train, and model proper body mechanics, I am on my way to success. In 2004, 70% of massage therapists quit work after three years because of work injuries! This is so sad and unfortunate.

The good news is that during my training program, we teach how to prevent injuries from happening! Seventy percent (70%) of the BodySmith training used in treatments are provided with body weight and elbows. Half of an hour providing Clinical Swedish Massage is used with fingers and the rest is used with relaxed knuckles and wrists.

In this guide, the very basics of body mechanics is touched on, but much more detail is involved in the actual training program. A good indicator that differentiates an experienced bodyworker from an unseasoned one is the awkwardness of pressure. If the practitioner is not comfortable with the technique, more than likely it's being done wrong and the client is aware of the awkwardness of the pose. A BodySmith moves around, maybe moves the client around, to adjust the technique thru the muscles adaptations (which are always changing)!

Staying grounded during a massage is critical. This grounding, or balancing includes having the skills to have one knee on the smithing table, the other leg standing on the stool, with an elbow/forearm evenly balanced with precise and almost perfect pressure (relating to the issue) on the serratus anterior or gluteus max, for example.

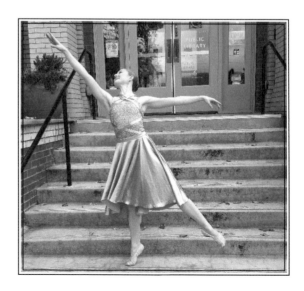

With this invisible horizontal line between the sun, you, and gravity, the BodySmither should be able to then perform passive and isolated resistance exercises, while pinning the muscle, paying attention to their own breathing in harmony with the clients, and being able to ride the wave of the muscles' adaptations.

Phew, so much is going on in this time and space. In comparison, a Surfer has perfect body mechanics. In the world, they are riding the waves of the ocean, waves that run in conjunction with the positioning of the moon! So here we are, BodySmiths riding the waves of the muscles that run in conjunction with neurons firing in the brain and central nervous system!

Are you convinced that how you treat your body tools are a critical reflection on your practice? Body mechanics is a delicate skill and necessary to facilitate the highest standard of care in bodysmithing.

A cheap unkept broken tool delivers poorly cared for material. An abused, uncared for, unhealthy massage therapist will deliver those results in their practice. Choosing to invest in well-kept tools will provide understanding, knowledge, and skill to come alongside a BodySmith and help improve a person's quality of life. To help equip the smith with great tools, I suggest taking a body mechanics and a sports massage class or even choose to study Rolfing.

Body Mechanics are cleverly woven in for both the smith and the client, as each works with the other. Proper bolstering for the client means their muscles are as close as they can be to a relaxed state. If this doesn't happen, we may think a stretched muscle is Hypertonic when it's not. Also, the BodySmith's extremities must work in between hyper-flexion and hyper-extension to maintain performance with the least stress put on their own body.

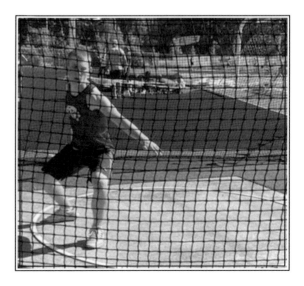

It's said a good name is better than great riches. Who is looking at you? What are people saying behind your back? Are most of your clients' referrals? Are you taking responsibility outside of the session to improve your quality of life? If you are doing your due diligence to stay healthy, you can be an encouragement to someone that's earnestly looking to improve their quality of life. I ask you, why anyone would not want to be healthy. To enjoy life and be able to help improve another person's quality of life gives one great purpose. Be it your spouse, your grandchildren, your community... We are all in this together.

Masks

Infamous 2020, the year that stole smiles, hugs, handshakes, travels and much more. A year turned upside to shake out the chaff. However, in 2021, while so any saw the times as falling apart, here at the BodySmith, we saw the times and pieces falling into place.

When many people saw the glass half empty, the idea of mask wearing was actually a glass half full for the BodySmith. The smith could now breathe while positioned over a client's upper body *without turning their head*. Besides saving the client from our fish breath, for those who have slipped disks or pinched nerves in the neck, the mildest flexion or extension of the neck could take a body worker out of commission!

The good news; along with proper body mechanics, the mask is a seat belt for your neck! All BodySmiths wear a mask to reflect the care for themselves (muscles, vertebrae and disks), so that in Infamous 2020, the year that stole smiles, hugs, handshakes, travels and much more. A year turned upside to shape this ever changing world, the client can have one less thing to think about.

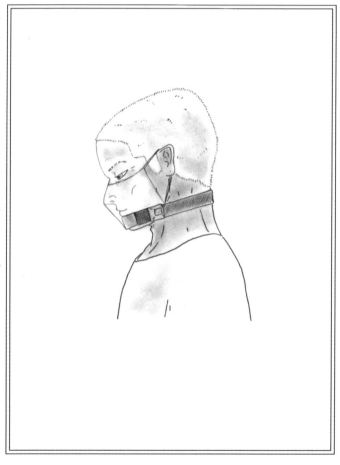

Pressure Scale

Pain that feels SO Good! Yes, this is what differentiates the seasoned from the unseasoned bodyworker. This philosophy is in complete contrast to the old fashioned moto of 'No pain, no gain.' At the BodySmith training program, the idea of what type of pain is acceptable in a massage is very scientific.

God created us with an amazing ability to deal with pain. In ancient caveman days, if a person was attacked, their flight (parasympathetic) or fight (sympathetic) response kicked in. A person would run or fight!

If in danger or injured, the human is designed for self-preservation and will move to escape a life threatening situation and pain. We hear about these stories all the time. Putting it simply, our adrenal glands, when put into a dire situation of flight or fight, stop the sensation of pain momentarily from registering in the brain. This is why a person who has been in a terrible car accident, full of shreds of glass, dazed and confused can get out of the vehicle, walk a short distance and hail for help. After about 15 min, the adrenal hormones become exhausted and a person will fall to the ground, cry out, and then pass out in severe pain.

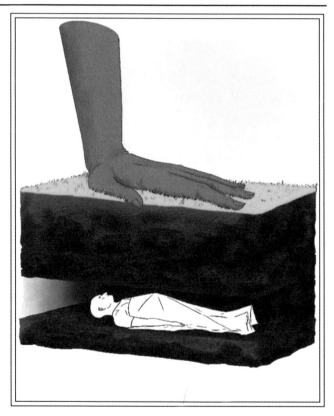

Ever heard of a person who received a 'Deep Tissue' massage and felt worse the next day or days afterwards? So much worse that they don't ever go back for bodywork again. This is not an ideal situation. For the BodySmith, the focus is on Pressure, NOT pain.

Our bodies are made of organic material similar to diamonds. Diamonds are created under immense pressure. Correct pressure creates the desired change and that can be implied in many settings.

Observation indicates that in many massage schools, people graduate with just enough knowledge to hurt someone. Of course clients will feel better when an uneducated body worker gets off the muscle. They were never doing it right in the first place!

This is why the BodySmith, with less than 2.5 years of practice and with 1000 hours of client time cannot use or get paid for using our treatment techniques. This is staying consistent with the standard and level of care taught in our training program. Perfect Pressure is acquired through time and experience.

By the way, there is a very small percentage of clients who want nothing other than to feel pain. I will refer them out after the first session. This is a psychological issue that needs to be addressed in a different setting outside the BodySmith training. Energy should not be spent on this type of pain in this practice. This heretic train of thought and practice falls short of all science and does more damage to the body than actually helps it.

This progressive and practical guide will teach BodySmiths to lean on the scientifically physiological quantitative data of pressure and the pain response in the brain, before they begin any treatment program. This practice increases the standard by which insurance companies will pay massage therapists to do the correct job.

Through personal experience, learning beside Dr. Zeyna Wine (a Russian medical doctor) and under a certified Rolfer who taught Sports treatment, I have derived the best, most efficient pressure scale. The BodySmith can acquire a miraculous way to reach a pressure threshold, scientifically aligned that improves a person's quality of life. A good testimony, shouting out a good job well done, is worth the time and energy spent teaching the BodySmith philosophy for Pain that feels so good.

Pressure Scale:

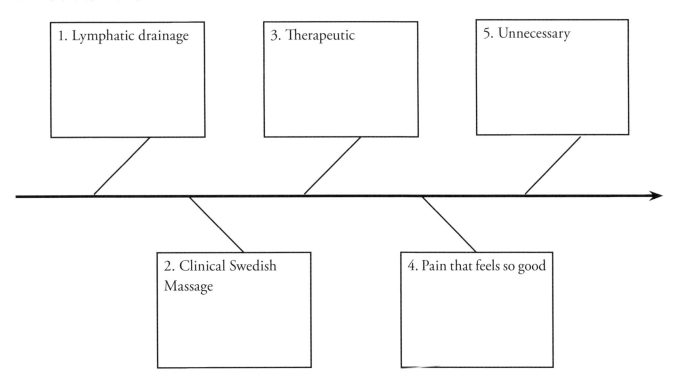

PART II:

MASSAGE AND TREATMENTS

Introducing the fun part of the book, this is where four sections are dedicated to unique and special massage techniques: Clinical Swedish, Therapeutic, Treatment and Side Lying. Each, on their own, contains a beauty that deserves special attention. Bodysmithing articulates each stroke to meet a varying need in each individual technique.

Aren't there more than four message techniques that are effective? Yes! Absolutely! However, in the journey of bodysmithing, so far, I have only been called to treat people in a practical and progressive way using these four modalities. In the latter part of the book, I touch on the human spirit which drives the effectiveness and longevity of bodysmithing. That section is So fun revealing our Temple!

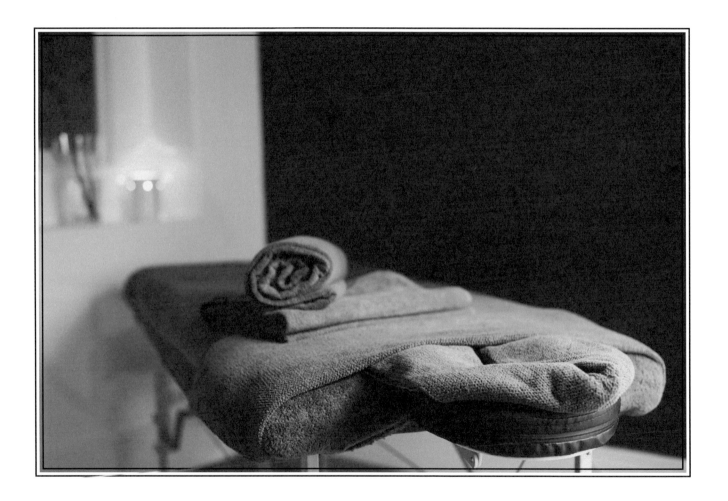

Clinical Swedish Massage

A car generally needs to get an oil changed every 3000 miles to run efficiently. If this is not done, the car will eventually run out of oil and a waterfall of catastrophes will ensue. Clinical Swedish Massage is the most basic of bodysmithing techniques, an 'oil change' for the body per say. The idea for this technique, while not SPA appropriate, is to decrease the sympathetic nervous system from firing and reduce pain perception.

Relaxation, could be the goal in this massage, but the main intention for bodysmithing purposes is Clinical. Nobody goes to the car wash, and leaves thinking the oil was changed. In fact, you could get a car wash and leave depressed if you knew the oil still needed changing. However, if you went and also got the oil changed, you would leave with peace of mind knowing you took care of the car's internal need.

Another analogy that can be applied to this Swedish technique is when buying an expensive piece of furniture, appliance, or outfit. If you pay in cash, the BodySmith way, it is yours forever, no strings attached. Paid in full. Done. If you pay for it with a credit card, you are still making payments for a while, paying interest, and technically it isn't yours free and clear.

The purpose of Clinical Swedish Massage for the BodySmith is maintaining a healthy body using four different strokes. Whenever investing in this type of massage, you are serving the body, mind and soul with something that cannot be taken away.

For health maintenance, this massage should be on everyone's calendar at least once a month. This is also the least expensive of all the massages and the modalities used are more soothing for a stressed person, and more stimulating for the tired person, making it a popular choice.

Techniques used to begin this massage are Effleurage and Petrissage; brother and sister. Effleurage is used to spread the lubricant. The intention of this stroke sets the stage for the massage. Since it is a Clinical Swedish Massage, generally, the stroke being an introductory or closing technique is very light. Muscle tone is usually not palpable here, but the speed of effleurage is usually determined on whether or not the person is stressed or distressed. The speeds of the stroke either quickly stimulate, or they are slow to soothe. In the psyche part of this guide, Core Insights, we will discuss the benefits of discerning a person's attitude, emotions, and body language to determine how a BodySmith will create an incredible session of healing.

Petrissage (IMO) is the best feeling of all the modalities in the Clinical Swedish Setting. It uses varying compressions of short strokes that depend on the muscle tissue. Firm pressure may be appropriate in some areas of high muscle hypertonicity, but it is the rhythmically consistent flow that is overall so helpful. There are 6 modalities within this service that are discussed more in detail within the BodySmith training program. Although, a few are mentioned in the later part of this guide.

The third technique in the Clinical Swedish Massage method is Vibration or Rocking. To imagine the benefits of the Vibration technique, pretend you are a little child. It's nighttime and you are scared. Grandma comes in and picks you up, carries you over to the rocking chair and rocks you until you have calmed down. Or, look at a crying baby. Its mother soothes it by gently rocking it until the baby falls asleep. Subconsciously, our body responds positively to the motion of vibration. On a side note, EMDR is another secular type of therapy that aligns itself with the idea of tapping into the subconscious for a deeper sense of healing and wellness.

Understand this, while we as BodySmiths work alongside a person, we are also aware that a person's quality of life depends on more than just wonderfully working muscles. Our craft is perfected when we can help the client, help themselves understand the full capabilities they possess for their wellness.

The fourth and most enjoyable of the four modalites is Tapotement. This is where we get to be drummers and bring to the smithing table a bit of native healing. Tapotement pushes down quickly on the skin multiple times over an area and the body pushes back with blood and muscle. Hence, this push and pull is restoring blood into the muscle.

The foundation to Clinical Swedish Massage is the consistent rhythmic strokes that are used with the four modalities; Effleurage, Petrissage (kneading), Vibration, and Tapotement. When applied the BodySmith way, this common massage creates a lasting change to the overall body.

Therapeutic Massage

Therapeutic massage is a full body deep pressure massage. This is the prominent difference between Clinical Swedish and Therapeutic massages. It must also be noted that deep pressure is not deep tissue. Touch Physiology, on its own, studies depths of pressure and effects on the central nervous system. Since BodySmiths are not treating muscles on a level of damage in a series (such as motor vehicle accidents), but evoking a deeper sense of relaxation and muscle release, we aim to keep deep tissue methods limited to Treatment Massage.

Many spas, chiropractic offices and clients refuse to accept the difference between deep pressure and deep tissue. However, still clarify this to every client and never do deep tissue straight for 90, 60, 30, and not even for 15 minutes. Refer clients out if that is what they are looking for, as the BodySmith way is not the path for them. True deep tissue focuses mainly on site specific areas for a longer time with a different prerogative in mind. This is discussed further in the next chapter detailing Treatment Massage.

The purpose of therapeutic body work is muscular, along with helping decrease the sympathetic nervous system and increase the parasympatheic nervous system. In elementary terms, therapeutic massage taps into our fight and flight response. BodySmiths address adhesions, trigger points, hypertonic muscles, use heat and cold, and stretch fascia for a greater pressure response.

Basically, the same four strokes are used as in a Swedish massage, but for therapeutic reasons, deeper pressure is applied. This body work begins with the introduction of a hot pack placed over the spine, opening the capillaries in the upper body, and drawing more blood to the surface, quicker than a slow manual stroking touch. Hence, a quicker, deeper, more intense sense of wellbeing.

Therapeutic massage would be most appropriately given by a journeyman in the BodySmith school second year of practice. And, for the client who is tired and has low energy, a Therapeutic massage will leave them with a stronger lasting impression.

Treatment Massage

Bam! Boom! BadaBing! A BodySmith shines in this ring. All of our experience, knowledge, and credibility is attributed to the ability to discern what a person is saying, how they are saying it, and what their body is displaying. Often a person will come in for a massage with pain in a particular area and the BodySmith will touch another area that is then determined to be the primary source of their pain. For example, pin and stretch the SITS MM's and the pecs loosen up or the ear unplugs! It's fascinating!

Real, quantitative research can be done here and clients can see and attest to improvement within three treatments. Rolfing is very similar and the philosophy Ida Rolf came up with almost aligns like the big dipper with the little dipper. However BodySmithers differ in our progressive approach. The conglomeration of the master pressure scale, Russian Medical, all mentioned techniques, and direct interaction with the clients, make these worth their money in gold.

Treatment massage with Deep Tissue is widely used for the purpose and primary goal of altering structures and muscle restriction with less emphasis on pleasure. Techniques are directly related to a site specific area, in a series of treatments to improve a person's wellness. The testimonies speak for themselves.

BodySmiths introduce Passive and Active Isolated Resistance along with vibration and GTO releases with the client's direct interaction. These techniques reduce muscle spasm and tone. Walking alongside the client takes them on their own journey to health. Similar to physical therapy they control the extent of sensation in the muscle movement. We coach them verbally, usually to use smaller movements, but overall, they drive the car.

We know that physiologically our bodies are stimulated by mechanical stimulations. Many tissues in our body have receptors that trigger the nervous system to react either positively or negatively. Hence, exposing the absolute farce in 'No pain No gain' philosophy. According to Zhenya Wine and her Russian Medical Massage book, the energy created by pressure applied to the body, along with movement sends signals to the CNS, exciting vasodilation or vasoconstriction, increased elasticity of fascia, possible release of hormones oxytocin, endorphins, acetylcholine, and more. The fact that we can scientifically explain so much of what goes on in a Treatment massage is why I love this work. With greater understanding, a BodySmith in their third year of schooling would be called a Novice and be more experienced to give these deep tissue Treatment massages.

Side-Lying Massage

Massage is so boring' – 'How do I fill in a two hour massage' – 'My client just isn't getting any better' - 'Side Lying is only for pregnant women'– 'yada, yada, yada'. I promise that when a client finds a BodySmith who is not afraid to use Side- Lying, they will have found a pot of Gold. The purpose is to include another dimension of body work through the knowledge of tensegrity. Without this knowledge, the therapist still lives and works in the box, no matter how 'intuitive' they may be.

Imagine putting on a vest. If the vest is too small you cannot put your arms into it. Too many laissez faire massage therapists work only the front and back. This is inside the box. When you open your minds, you will see that the sides of the body are not being taken care of like the front and the back. They will pull the muscles right back to where a person started from. What a waste of time!

The BodySmith knows their time is valuable and want that relayed with the effectiveness of their treatments. When they get paid, the client's testimony should match their cost. That's when the smith leaves the session with a sense of personal satisfaction knowing their hard work helped their client.

Side-Lying massage is not just for pregnant women. It's effective in treatment with larger clients and kids too. We are not disturbing a client's 'Zens' by rolling them over or asking them to gently push and pull certain muscles while treating their upper, mid or low back. In fact, they feel more involved in their health. Interactive treatments are often taken outside, into the real world where they *intentionally* make their investment become their own. What a great practice the BodySmith has with testimonies from their clients claiming victory with what they have left their sessions with. Peace of mind and assurance that they can take care of themselves and their bodies. This is all achieved from Side-Lying Massage.

Mastering the Side-Lying skill increases clientele (mostly through word of mouth), awakens proprioceptors that ignite the CNS (making the effort worthwhile), and generates better quality healthcare. Treatment overall is the objective unless one is pregnant or heavier set.

Knowing the tensegrity of the human body is imperative to being an incredible, talked about, searched for BodySmith. It differentiates the apprentice from the novice. The bottom line is that most clients would prefer to spend their time, efforts, and cash on someone who knows what they are doing. That is what they get with the everyday BodySmith.

Knowledge, combined with research and hundreds of hours of experience make credible distinctions between BodySmiths and other bodyworkers.

Simple TX

These two basic treatments, Upper and Lower Body Techniques, will also differentiate the everyday BodySmith from other body workers. Please remember these are simple treatments and only produce outcomes based on real people with individual needs. Everyone will be different, but these methods will be similar.

On the following pages, two sample treatment sessions are illustrated.

Upper Body Treatment Techniques
Pictures taken in the BodySmith Studio.

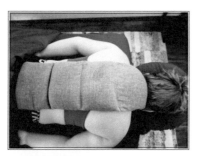

Begin the session with Hot Pack placed along the ESG's, Paraspinals and between shoulder blades. Either Pin and stretch the gluteal muscles, or begin with foot massage. 10 Min max.

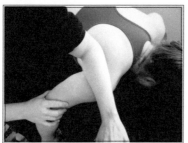

Using appropriate body mechanics and leverage, MFR, Deep Tissue, Deep Pressure, and PIR/AIR (in directions that needed most) are used on Teres Major and Lats (complete synergists) and Rotator Cuff muscles: Supra, infra, teres minor, subscap.

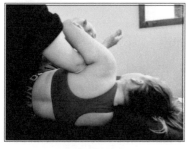

Side-Lying, Deep Pressure, PIR/AIR MFR with forearms and proper body mechanics (using a stool if necessary). Lats posterior to spinous process of last 6 thoracic vertebrae, last 3 or 4 ribs, Subscapularis, Serratus Anterior and External oblique.

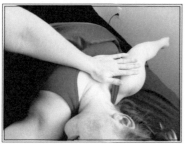

Client lying in Prone position, MFR Pec major, p/s serratus anterior, Pec minor, GTO release, Supraspinatus, infraspinatus along Greater Tubercle of humerus, Deltoid post and med. Gentle kneading upper fibers trapezius and cervical muscles.

Lower Body Treatment Techniques

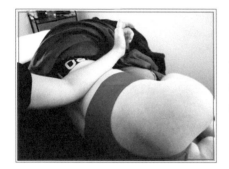

Hot pack horizontally placed along Iliac crest, Side-Lying, Gluteal fascia, external obliques, Lats. MFR, Gliding, Deep Pressure, PIR/AIR, forearms and elbow and above muscles including Psoas major and minor.

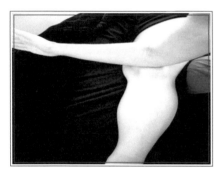

Client laying prone, PIR/AIR, MFR, Deep Pressure over ASIS & AIIS, proper body mechanics, forearms, elbow Sartorius, TFL, Rectus Femoris, Vastus Lateralis. DT, PIR/AIR Rectus Femoris, Vastus Med and Lateralis above the Tibial Tuberosity.

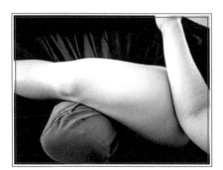

Direct Pressure, head of fibula on bicep femoris, PIR/AIR, DP kneading with knuckles, Peronius Longus, Brevis, Soleus, Gastroc, along with Tibia Anterior and Flexors.

PART III:

CORE INSIGHTS

Where it all Begins Matters. Are you Equipped for Battle? Is Your Temple Protected?

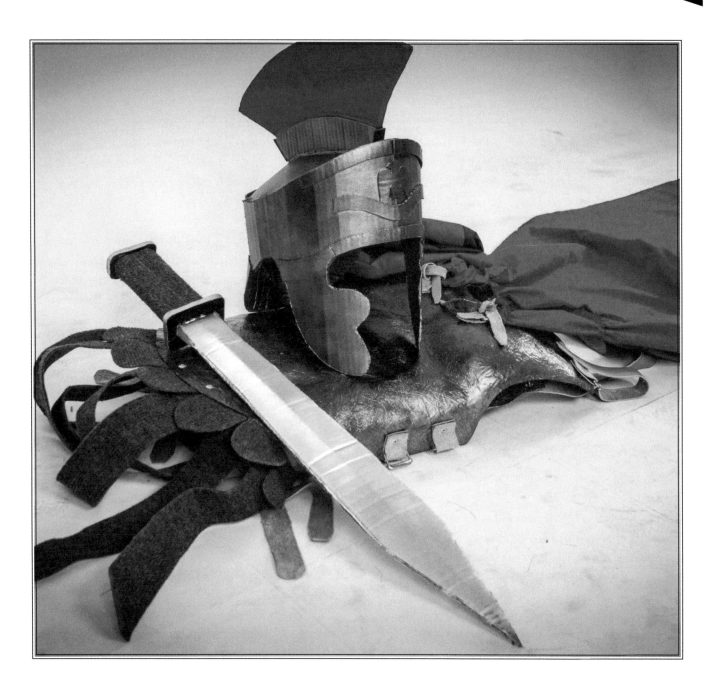

Body-Armor

After 16 years of bodysmithing, I have discerned that everyone wears some type of invisible Armor. People are unaware of this protection, neglecting to maintain its function; to protect them. This can be seen in the muscles, how a person treats their self. The Armor is similar to what a Roman soldier wears; the belt, the breastplate, the shoes, the helmet, the shield, and the sword. Briefly, I will share how this is seen through my eyes and processed through my practice.

While working on someone's shoulder girdle, I think to myself that their breastplate needs a refit. I rearrange a few things (muscular and facially) enabling better range of motion, decreasing pain, with the intention of seeing a whole person, not just the muscle.

Lower back and abdominals help me visualize a person's belt Armor. I ask myself, is it too tight? Is it too loose? Is one side hiked up or forward? The belt in a Roman's Armor holds together the breastplate and the sword. If this area of a person is not in balance with the natural way their body should be, the other two parts it holds together will suffer.

Analyzing a person's gate and walk shows me if the shoes are fitted wrong. Or, perhaps they are wearing the wrong kind of shoes for the 'battle' they are in. Are the feet outwardly turned or do they walk bow legged?

All observations are seen through this lens and it has profound effects on the energy that is produced in the treatments. Let's take the shackles off our feet so we can dance.

The neck and facial distortions are often related to a crooked or miss-fitting helmet. Can a football player perform at their best if the helmet doesn't fit perfectly? The same concept fits for our invisible helmet that protects our thoughts, stamina, intention, delivery, speech, and attitude.

The shield held onto by the hand gives me pause when working a person's forearms, hands and fingers. Is their grip because of the job they do or maybe from worry or concern? The hands along with the feet have been anciently observed and reflexology has become the result. This is not something I put much thought into, but worth noting.

The sword is the only thing a person can use to fight with. Honestly, looking at this piece of Armor helps to see if a person is willing to be intentional about their health journey. How much are they willing to cut bad habits, change their lifestyle to get better or invest in themselves, are the questions to ask. Remember, the BodySmith's motto is 'to help improve your quality of life.' We don't 'fix' your muscular problems. We walk alongside you on your own health journey and discovery.

We want you to live your best life continuously. We don't want to see the same person for the same thing year after year. We improve our own skills for your future.

Is a positive outlook on life with a desire to grow in knowledge and understanding of your body the sword you use? Do you realize that being in control of your health gives you great power? Being proactive with your health and how the body works, most always keeps you alive longer and living a better quality of life.

After I finish every session, I find great satisfaction when a person feels they are fitted more properly for battle when they walk out the door. Hopefully, they won't continue habits that got them where they were and will awaken from a slumber that was brought on by Armor so wrongly fitted, where true blood circulation could not occur. Remember, blood moves oxygen throughout the body and transports all types of cells to their designated job. Our bodies like to do their job naturally.

When a client leaves a session with confidence, knowing that they now have this knowledge, the investment is not in vain. Sometimes, we need new screws, metal strips, an oil up on hinges, help with fastening hooks or laces. I hope this BodySmith Armor train of thought encourages you to also remain steadfast on your own health journey. Half the battle is just showing up. You got this and so do we!

Put on

THE FULL ARMOR OF GOD

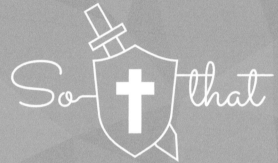

So that

YOU CAN TAKE YOUR STAND
AGAINST THE DEVIL'S SCHEMES

Ephesians 6:11

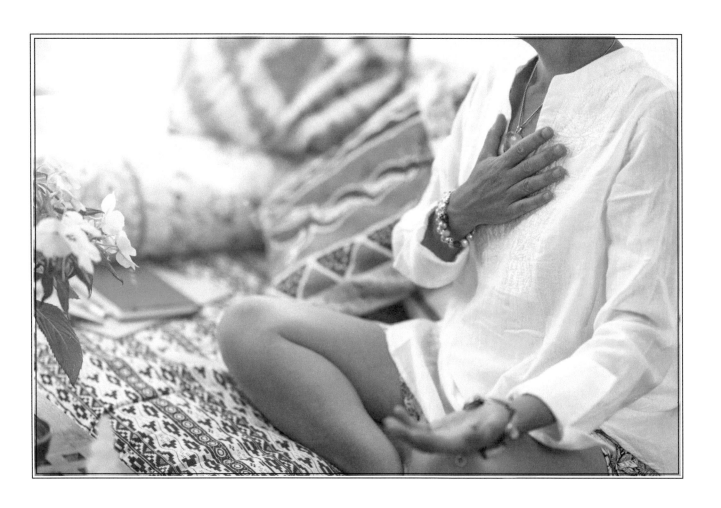

The Temple

What is spiritual disorder? What is physical disorder? How does spiritual disorder contribute to bodily physical disorder? Why is it imperative to put on spiritual body Armor and how can we wear it effectively to take care of our physical body? Bodysmithing is a spiritual gift. In this guide, I am addressing physical disorders, wants, and needs, while paying close attention to spiritual elements as they coincide with the Bible.

People already 'awake' to this spiritual basis only need maintenance on their Armor (physically and spiritually). Overall, they are good caretakers of the 'temple' they live in. Some people are still asleep and hardly see the correlation between what disorder their body is in and the true spiritual disorder their soul is in. These folks rarely benefit longer than a day from bodysmithing, always wanting more, feeding another physical need without realizing their need for 'spiritual water'.

Some people are 'lukewarm' understanding their physical disorder can be tempered with the right mindset or habit change. The idea of 'armoring up' makes sense, but in general, their condition is manageable and little change is done due to comfortability of circumstance.

What types of spiritual disorders are there? To name a several, sadness or depression (chemical imbalance), gluttony, selfish ambition, loose tongue or a gossiper, stiffnecked, proud, discontentment, attention issues, bitter, and angery.

How do these spiritual disorders contribute to physical disorder? With sadness also comes racing thoughts, anxiety, confusion, defeat and it can manifest into 'Clinical Depression.' Physical disorders can be seen in lethargy and weight gain from prescription drugs and bone density loss from the use of street drugs (often used to escape the reality that seriously concerns the individual).

Gluttony disorder is seen obviously in the mid-section of the body. Having a loose middle causes severe stress on the back muscles used to stabilize a person when they stand up. Physically, this also contributes to food and digestion issues.

The spiritual disorders of selfish ambition, being a gossiper, stiff-necked and proud, all result in headaches, neck stiffness, and vertebral disorders such as degenerative disk disease, or bulging disks in the upper cervical region.

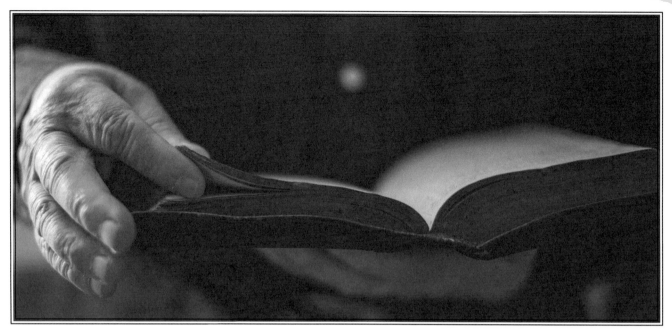

Spiritual discontentment and attention issues lead to physical pain that is not actually a muscle thing that can be completely helped with bodysmithing. That becomes a generalized full body feeling of pain, for example Fibromyalgia comes to mind. Escaping the firing of the body nerve endings is mentally exhausting and can lead to medication and a slant on reality. Physically, the BodySmith can do little except bring minimal relief for a person, for a very short period of time. Here, the mind absolutely needs to change before the body can.

Two final spiritual disorders to mention are bitterness and anger. These present themselves in the body as very tight, short, hardened muscles. Muscles are so tight that they can impinge nerves causing numbing and a tingling down the arm or down the leg. Sometimes a person needs the pressure to hurt before they say

they can fully relax. People hide behind the 'no pain no gain' mentality here. Muscles feel fused together with little flexibility or range of motion being present. Physically and spiritually, this person is a challenge to work with.

So, if having a physical need is connected to a spiritual need, why is it important to 'armor up'? What is armoring up? It is a spiritual discipline every person who wants to lead healthy, effective, productive lives must do. A war is going on in the spiritual realm we don't physically see and as spiritual people, I believe we all must protect ourselves in this spiritual warfare. Our spiritual weapons, found in reading and applying bible scripture, can defeat the enemy who wants to destroy us physically, mentally, emotionally and spiritually. Do not let him hurt you. Armor up and get ready to fight for your best life ever.

DISCLAIMER:

While the Holy Bible provides answers on how to take care of our body, and why we should do so, I want to also put a disclaimer in this book. While I faithfully use the Bible as a guide in bodysmithing, to help folks obtain and sustain a good quality of life, sometimes there are cases I cannot help or even understand. This is how life goes sometimes. Everything is credited to the God I serve, Jesus Christ. He does the healing, I just show up armed and ready to be a vessel of His healing power. Sometimes, He chooses not to heal and His reasons I don't have to understand. I just trust that His purposes prevail and He does win the war in the end.

Case in point, there is an incredible story of a man named Job in the Bible. Job was 'blameless and upright, a man who feared God and shunned evil' (Job 1:8). Satan, the adversary of every person past, present and future, came to present himself before the Lord and asked to strike everything Job had, to show God that surely Job would 'curse you to your face' (Job 1:11). God *ALLOWED* satan to steal his property, burn his sheep and servants, his sons and daughters all died after a mighty wind collapsed the building in which they all were under. God allowed satan to afflict Job with loathsome sores and even Job's wife accused him of doing something that CAUSED all of this.

Sometimes, our health, family relationships, and adversity in the workplace have more to do with our integrity, than they do with understanding what the heck is going on. Job was unaware of the heavenly activity behind his circumstances and sometimes we are too. That's why this disclaimer is here. Sometimes, we cannot fix what is going on in our body, family or work. But we must be well armored spiritually to withstand the schemes of the evil one, while Life sometimes has no rhyme or reason. As a BodySmith, I try to help, but if that's not the Will of God, it won't happen.

I am a follower of Jesus, and believe His power is at work through the Holy Spirit that lives in me. There is no spirit as powerful and mighty as the One involved with the Trinity. I believe in His saving power, along with His healing power. Not everyone working in the BodySmith training program has these same values as myself. As a praying person who's been given this desire to share this informative, philosophy driven, practical and progressive guide, I want you the reader to know that any help that comes from my practice was ordained by someone much more powerful than myself or anyone working alongside me. May you be blessed and healed thru any BodySmith in Jesus Name!

ACKNOWLEDGEMENTS

A thanks for the following:

Travis Lundberg, Mercy Johnston, Nate Santon   page 7

Jared Isaac   page 9,

Angela Schroeder   page 10

Mercy Johnston   page11

River Myers, illustrator of Seatbelt man   page13

Diamond man   page 14

Patience Johnston (model)   page 25-26

Patience and Mercy Johnston

Printed in the United States
by Baker & Taylor Publisher Services

Printed in the United States
By Bookmasters